Legal & Disclaimer

The information contained in this book and its contents is not designed to replace or take the place of any form of medical or professional advice; and is not meant to replace the need for independent medical, financial, legal or other professional advice or services, as may be required. The content and information in this book have been provided for educational and entertainment purposes only.

You agree that by continuing to read this book, where appropriate and/or necessary, you shall consult a professional (including but not limited to your doctor, attorney, or financial advisor or such other advisor as needed) before using any of the suggested remedies, techniques, or information in this book.

TABLE OF CONTENTS

INTRODUCTION

Unless you have been living under a rock for the past few years, you will likely have heard of The Paleo Diet, Paleolithic nutrition, or the hunter-gatherer diet to describe a way of eating that mimics the diet of our ancestral past.

The basic argument for following this way of eating is that, for the majority of humanity's time on this earth, this is how we ate, and it subsequently shaped our genetics. This is particularly the case in terms of how we, as humans, respond to the foods we eat, to the prevention of disease, and the vitality of our species.

While there has been a massive change in the food supply—starting with the agricultural revolution 10,000 years ago, then, the advent of dairy farming 5,000 years ago, and the more recent industrial revolution— our genetic makeup has not kept pace with these accelerated changes in our food supply. While humans do adapt, as in the case of some recent genetic mutations such as the adult lactase persistence(ALP) gene, these changes take place extremely slowly, resulting in an incongruence between our physiology and the foods eaten on a typical modern diet in the Western world.

The paleo diet is a great choice no matter whether you're looking to kickstart your New Year's goals or just want to live a healthier, clean eating lifestyle. This paleo for beginners guide will help you learn the ins and outs of the paleo diet, complete with everything you need to know about getting started with paleo.

This is the diet of our hunter-gatherer ancestors. It comprises the basic foods eaten by every human since our first appearance over a million years ago, until the invention of agriculture a mere 10,000 years ago. Of course, many of the foods that ancestral man consumed no longer exist. Therefore, the modern Paleo Diet mimics the foods that we would have consumed in our historic past. It is as close as we can get to a diet unadulterated by modern agricultural methods, animal husbandry, or processed foods, elements that have only existed for a short amount of time relative to the span of human evolution.

If you're looking to feel healthier and more energetic, here are the paleo for beginners guidelines you need to know. You'll find answers to the most frequently asked questions about the paleo diet. You'll also find quick and easy paleo recipes to help fill your meal plan and get you started on the right foot. So you can skip all of the overwhelm and get started with healthy eating success.

WHAT IS THE PALEO DIET?

The Paleo Diet focuses on a high-protein, low-carb plan, which emphasizes eating meat, fruits, and vegetables—basically, anything available to your Paleolithic ancestors 10,000 years ago.

Go Paleo and you'll have to cut out processed foods (primitives didn't have microwaves for frozen pizza), which probably isn't a surprise to you.

What will likely shock you is that people on the Paleo Diet shouldn't eat grains, legumes, dairy, potatoes, refined vegetable oils, and salt.

Although, you can put sabertooth tiger back on the menu, har har.

And you can do the same for grass-fed beef, seafood, fresh fruits and vegetables, eggs, nuts, and seeds. Specific oils including, coconut, avocado, and olive, are also Paleo-friendly.

A typical Paleo dinner could include grilled chicken with steamed vegetables and fruit for dessert.

Yeah, kind of crazy, right?

The Paleo Diet is a diet that intends to imitate the eating habits of our Palaeolithic ancestors. It is one that forms a radically different approach to traditional diets of today. Often referred to as the 'caveman' diet, it consists of foods that can be hunted, fished and gathered.

This ultimately includes:

1. Lean meat

2. Seafood

3. Fruits

4. Vegetables

The Paleo diet is also known as the hunter-gatherer diet due to the way food was obtained and consumed. Men would hunt wild animals and catch fish, while women would gather fruit, berries, nuts and vegetables. Agricultural systems had not been developed during this time period so grains were not in anyway a part of the caveman's diet. Much like all diets, it is used by individuals seeking to lose weight or live healthier as instead on focusing on foods that are simply convenient and tasty, greater importance is placed on foods containing minerals, vitamins and nutrients required for healthy bodily functioning.

Though there are many individuals who describe the Paleo diet as nothing more than another low-carb fad, there is some substantial scientific evidence backing its claims.

The basic argument for following this way of eating is that, for most of human history, it is how we ate, and it subsequently shaped our genetics.

This is particularly true in terms of how we, as humans, respond to the foods we eat, to the prevention of disease, and the vitality of our species. While there have been massive changes in the food supply—starting with the agricultural revolution 10,000 years ago, then, the advent of dairy farming 5,000 years ago, and the more recent industrial revolution—our genetic makeup has not kept pace.

Humans do adapt to changes. For example, the genetic mutation that led to the development of adult lactase persistence (ALP) - allowing some of us to digest lactose in milk into adulthood - took place very recently, from an evolutionary standpoint. But when looked at in terms of human generations, we actually adapt very slowly. This can result in an incongruence between our physiology and our environment. That is the case with the typical modern diet in the Western world. Over 70 percent of the foods we eat were introduced since our last major evolutionary change and we simply haven't caught up.

There are many nutritional advantages to following a more ancestral nutrient-rich diet comprised mainly of fresh fruits, fresh vegetables, fish, shellfish, grass produced meats and organ meats, free-range poultry, free-range eggs, nuts, and certain healthful oils.

The Paleo Diet avoids or eliminates processed foods containing refined sugars, refined grains, refined vegetable oils, trans fatty acids, salt, and added chemicals. Fresh fruits and fresh vegetables, good sources of healthier carbohydrates, are consumed ad libitum in lieu of refined sugars, refined grains, and processed foods. As a result, The Paleo Diet is a low glycemic load diet which promotes normalization of blood glucose, insulin, and helps prevent the metabolic syndrome.

In addition, the foods that constitute a modern Paleo Diet contain few problematic dietary anti-nutrients such as lectins, which can lead to a host of health concerns, including autoimmune diseases.

Ultimately, providing our physiology with foods that match our genetically determined nutritional requirements is why The Paleo Diet will provide you with long lasting health.

Theory Behind "The Paleo Diet"

The theory behind the Paleo diet lies essentially in the genetic makeup of human beings and the way it has evolved over the past 10,000 years. Scientists and researchers claim that the way humans utilise food, much like our genetic code, has changed very little over this period of time whilst new diseases and disease rates themselves have dramatically increased. Over this time period as well, human physiology has generally remained the same whilst environment and society have notably changed. This forms part of the theory why humans today require excellent healthcare systems, since the modern diet does in no way keep us healthy and strong.

Research findings have also provided sufficient evidence to state that these hunter-gatherer tribes were indeed very healthy; being taller, having better builds and bigger brains. Though their life expectancy was shorter, this was in large part due to external factors such as extreme weather conditions, predators and infections. Whereas modern man is now plagued with diseases such as diabetes, cancer and heart disease, our ancestors were not. These diseases are in large part a by product of human shift to agriculture; a 'mismatch' of our genetic components and our lifestyle.

The basic and most fundamental principle behind the Paleo diet is that the food our Palaeolithic ancestors consumed is still best suited for our bodies and metabolisms even today.

There are three primary reasons why the Palaeolithic diet formed a natural part of daily life for our ancestors. The first is that humans in that period were nearly always involved in physical activity as they hunted animals and actively sought out plants that would sustain them.

The plants that the Palaeolithic people consumed did also grow naturally in the wild. In comparison with today, they would have had a lower glycemic index (a measure of the quality of carbohydrates in comparison to the amount of total grams). Due to this lower glycemic index, the foods had a much less significant impact on insulin levels in their bloodstream than today's foods with their over processed starches and sugars. In all, this means that early humans could eat foods without the striking blood sugar highs and lows that people have when eating modern food.

The Paleo diet itself also encourages the consumption of grass-fed animals rather than grain-fed ones as it is believed they have less saturated fats that are the cause of many health problems today. Simply put, the idea is to have the leanest source of meat possible that the modern world has to offer.

Starter Tips: What Do I Need To Know?

When you're a paleo beginner you'll want to start with looking at what's in the foods you're currently eating. You may be surprised to find what's in the ingredients list!

I remember feeling like gluten, grains and refined sugars seemed to be hiding in practically everything I picked up. Of course, once you learn what to avoid and how to read your food labels it becomes so much easier to meal plan and grocery shop.

You'll want to stock your paleo pantry with compliant foods, so you have all the paleo ingredients on hand. You'll also want to grab your list of paleo foods to get you ready to shop for pantry and fridge staples. After you decide to go paleo, your first shopping trips will be focused on buying the ingredients you need right away, while also slowly building your supply of pantry staples over time. You'll quickly find that you'll be shopping the perimeter of your grocery store, spending a good chunk of time looking at whole foods in the produce, meat and seafood department.

Of course, not all whole foods are created equally. You'll want to focus on purchasing the highest-quality Ingredientsavailable. Buy fresh in-season produce, organic meats, and sustainable seafood whenever possible. I do try to buy organic produce, especially for the dirty dozen.

Shopping for healthy Ingredientscan be expensive, and, depending on where you're located, it can also be time-consuming to actually source compliant ingredients. If this is the case for you, there are great online alternatives to traditional grocery stores

HEALTH BENEFITS OF A PALEO DIET

For most people the fact the Paleo diet delivers the best results is all they need. Improved blood lipids, weight loss, and reduced pain from autoimmunity is proof enough.

Many people however are not satisfied with blindly following any recommendations, be they nutrition or exercise related. Some folks like to know WHY they are doing something. Fortunately, the Paleo diet has stood not only the test of time, but also the rigors of scientific scrutiny.

With a very simple shift we not only remove the foods that are at odds with our health (grains, legumes, and dairy) but we also increase our intake of vitamins, minerals, and antioxidants.

Here is a great paper from Professor Loren Cordain exploring how to build a modern Paleo diet: The nutritional characteristics of a contemporary diet based upon Paleolithic food groups. This paper also offers significant insight as to the amounts and ratios of protein, carbohydrate and fat in the ancestral diet.

Come on! Our Ancestors lived short, brutal lives! This Paleo Diet is all bunk, right?

The Paleo concept is new for most people and this newness can spark many questions. We like people to not only read about and educate themselves on this topic but also to "get in and do it."

Experience is perhaps the best teacher and often cuts through any confusion surrounding this way of eating.

Now, all that considered, there are still some common counter arguments to the Paleo diet that happen with sufficient frequency that a whole paper was written on it.

Individuals choose the Paleo diet for a vast variety of different reasons and in this way, one can expect differing results for each person. Those who do follow the diet strictly will tell you that it has improved their energy levels, bodies and mood as well as a whole host of other benefits. The most obvious benefit of taking up the Paleo diet is the fact that you are eating unprocessed, real foods that are likely to help you lose weight, and lose it fast. By eating these unprocessed foods, you automatically remove a whole list of nasties like preservatives, additives, artificial colouring and flavouring and god knows what else! As consequence, you eliminate toxins from your diet and allow your body to function at its finest, absorbing healthy vitamins, minerals and nutrients. On top of this – your food will taste so much better! In many ways adopting the Paleo diet really is a win-win situation.

Diabetes

A great question to ask is "Does the Paleo diet work?" Here we have a head to head comparison between the Paleo diet and Mediterranean diet in insulin resistant Type 2 Diabetics.

The results? The Paleo diet group REVERSED the signs and symptoms of insulin resistant, Type 2 diabetes. The Mediterranean diet showed little if any improvements.

It is worth noting that the Mediterranean diet is generally held up by our government as "the diet to emulate" despite better alternatives.

Cardio Vascular Disease

According to the CDC, cardiovascular disease is the number one cause of death in the United States. Interestingly however, our Paleolithic ancestors and contemporarily studied hunter-gatherers showed virtually no heart attack or stroke while eating ancestral diets.

Autoimmunity

Autoimmunity is a process in which our bodies own immune system attacks "us."

Normally the immune system protects us from bacterial, viral, and parasitic infections. The immune system identifies a foreign invader, attacks it, and ideally clears the infection.

A good analogy for autoimmunity is the case of tissue rejection after organ donation. If someone requires a new heart, lung kidney or liver due to disease or injury, a donor organ may be an option.

The first step in this process is trying to find a tissue "match". All of us have molecules in our tissues that our immune system uses to recognize self from non-self. If a donated organ is not close enough to the recipient in tissue type the immune system will attack and destroy the organ.

In autoimmunity, a similar process occurs in that an individuals own tissue is confused as something foreign and the immune system attacks this "mislabeled" tissue.

Common forms of autoimmunity include Multiple Sclerosis, Rheumatoid Arthritis, Lupus, and Vitiligo to name only a tiny fraction of autoimmune diseases. Elements of autoimmunity are likely at play in conditions as seemingly unrelated as Schizophrenia, infertility, and various forms of cancer.

High Protein

Studies of hunter-gatherer tribes and populates demonstrate that these people typically derived 45%-60% of their calories from animal food sources. Only 14% of these societies consumed more than 50% of their calories from plant sources. Although western diets, with their increased meat consumption have been associated with higher rates of cardiovascular diseases and cancer, it is odd that these Palaeolithic societies were relatively free from such disease.

One of the most notable aspects of a Paleo diet meal plan is that it will generally include a high level of protein. Though this is of course a good benefit (especially for athletes and bodybuilders) it should not distract you from the basic tenet behind the diet – that is to consume real, natural and unprocessed foods. A major benefit of eating a greater amount of protein is that it helps individuals stay full for longer. Proteins require significantly more time to break down in the gut than most other foods such as fruits and vegetables. In this way the paleo diet really is excellent for those looking to manage their weight as it will help prevent hunger pangs and thus you will consume fewer calories.

In addition to this, the flesh of wild game is roughly around 2-4% fat by weight and contains significantly high levels of monounsaturated fat as opposed to grain-fed meats which can contain anywhere from 20% to 30% of fat; much of it saturated and definitely unhealthy. It is not the amount of meat and protein that one should be observing when on the Paleo diet, but rather the composition, quality and cooking methods which really determine the health status of the food. Recent scientific studies seem to highlight the fact that meat consumption is not actually directly correlated with cardiovascular disease but rather it is the saturated fat typically found in the meat of most modern domesticated animals. Diets high in protein can be seen to improve lipid profiles and leads to what is known as the thermogenesis effect in the body whereby your metabolism is significantly boosted.

As already stated, you must not forget that cooking methods are too of vital importance as cooking red meats at high temperatures produces high levels of chemicals known as heterocyclic amines which have been implicated in the development of gastrointestinal and prostate cancer. Meats that are highly salted should also be avoided, not just because salt intake should be limited on the Paleo diet but because these preserved meats often can carcinogens. It is about maintaining the balance between lean fresh meat and a high intake of vegetables and fruits that will ultimately give you the results you are looking for.

The Good Fats

According to studies, monounsaturated fats constituted roughly half of all the total fat in the diets of most hunter-gatherer tribes. When substituted for digestible starches and sugars, mono-unsaturated fats have also shown to reduce the risk of cardiovascular disease. For any paleo-dieter, nuts (in moderation of course) are a vital source of monounsaturated fats and have demonstrated cardioprotective qualities in a number of studies. The calories in nuts are usually around 80% fat which is made up of monounsaturated and polyunsaturated fatty acids including Omega-3. Studies have demonstrated that regular consumption of nuts (aroundabout 5 times a week) is associated with a 50% reduction in the risk of myocardial infarction. The benefits of consuming nuts on a regular basis also extend to lowered risk of type-2 diabetes, lower LDL (bad cholesterol) without having a negative effect on HDL (good cholesterol).

The paleo diet is one that as much as being high in protein, does not neglect your primary source of energy which in this case is fat. Eating lean meat that is sourced from grass-fed animals also means that the food you eat is high in good quality fat yet low in unhealthy saturated fats. The Paleo diet also allows individuals to get monounsaturated healthy fat from other sources such as poultry, seafood, ghee and coconuts. Monounsaturated fats are essential for healthy arteries, brain function as well as reducing systemic inflammation.

Eliminating processed foods from your diet will also inevitably to a dramatic decline in the amount of trans-fats you consume which contribute to conditions such as coronary heart disease. Trans-fatty acids are also found in most margarines and deep-fried foods and additionally in canola oil. They are known to lower HDL levels and increase LDL levels leading to an increased risk of cardiovascular disease and cancer. Some studies have indicated that just by simply replacing trans-fats (which constitutes about 2% of the total calories in an American diet) with the same amount of monounsaturated fats could lead to a 50% decrease risk of developing coronary heart disease.

Low in Carbohydrates

The amount of carbohydrates one can consume on the Paleo diet is quite low, very low in fact. The idea behind this is that the carbs we consume today (which usually come from grains, corn and legumes) were not available during the Stone Age. Those carbohydrates which were consumed during that time period also possessed a low glycemic load, meaning they released energy slowly and steadily to our Palaeolithic ancestors. By mimicking them, what we essentially do is not only take on their behaviours, but take on the positive effects they would have felt from eating such a diet. For example, low-carb diets have shown to aid in weight loss and prevent cravings for refined (processed) unhealthy carbohydrates you find in sugary snacks and drinks. This in essence defeats hunger pangs and prevents binge eating.

If you suffer from high blood pressure, adopting a low-carb diet is also a good idea as it has shown in some studies to lower blood pressure. Additionally, in a world that suffers from seemingly out-of-control rates of certain diseases such as diabetes, a low-carb diet is generally seen as a way of both treating this condition as well as preventing it. Low-carb diets reduce LDL (bad cholesterol) and increase HDL (good cholesterol) and in some cases can leave an individual feeling much more energetic.

Vitamins, Nutrients & Minerals

Nearly everyone today supplements some vitamin or mineral yet our Palaeolithic ancestor's did obviously not have access to modern medicine and supplements. This of course doesn't mean you should stop supplementing anything you are already currently taking. However what it does highlight is that many of the practices we have today were non-existent back then yet still the remains of our cavemen ancestors do not show any signs of the diseases that exist in the modern world. This is simply because the Paleo diet in many ways can account for virtually all other nutritional requirements.

With the Paleo diet you are will naturally be consuming high amounts of fruits and vegetables meaning you will get your RDA (Recommended Daily Allowance) of key vitamins and minerals. Green leafy vegetables such as spinach and broccoli contain high levels of vitamin K and iron. Olive oil, which is used in cooking by many paleo-dieters is also high in Vitamin E which is excellent for the skin. Fruits such as oranges are high in Vitamin C – you really are completely covered!

In addition to this, eating a good amount of fish will also mean that you will consume a good proportion of Omega-3 fatty acids. Those who do not enjoy eating fish would do well instead to consume plenty of avocado which in addition to containing healthy fatty acids also provides Vitamin E, B, potassium and fiber. The amount of fiber you consume while on the Paleo diet should be also be relatively high. This is mainly because you will be eating fruits, nuts, vegetables, and berries which are excellent sources of it. This fiber content is not only useful in the maintenance of bowel health, but also is connected to better levels of insulin as well as reduced risk of developing certain cancers. The fiber you consume, alongside sufficient levels of water will also reduce the bloating feeling (and physical effect!) that many people have when eating a standard Western diet. Additionally the paleo diet also help to improve the flora in your gut which is pivotal in maintaining a healthy digestive system.

Since you are not going to be consuming any processed foods, you thereby also dramatically decrease your salt intake. While this means your sodium intake will be reduced, your potassium levels should remain rather high – such diets which are low in sodium and high in potassium have time and time again demonstrated themselves to help alleviate chronic conditions such as hypertension and osteoporosis.

Insulin Response

If you suffer from fluctuating blood sugar levels or diabetes, the Paleo diet is bound to improve your insulin response. This is because the glycemic index of foods on the Paleo diet is much lower than most of the food people eat today. The glycemic index basically shows insulin response in the body when a certain food is eaten. It is a well-known fact that lean meats certain vegetables and nuts are low on the glycemic index. Although the diet does recommend eating fruit which is high in sugar content, it still possesses a lower glycemic load than the refined sugars and carbohydrates found in soft drinks and other processed foods.

Beverages

While on the Paleo diet, you will of course be imitating the habits of early humans, and this too includes what you drink. Our Palaeolithic ancestors drank pretty much water only. Recent findings demonstrate that 5 or more glasses of water a day can lower your risk of developing coronary heart disease. The reasoning behind this is not fully clear with some arguing that is detoxifying the body by removing calorie-dense drinks (sodas etc.) and others stating that it provides sufficient hydration to reduce blood viscosity. Whatever the reason behind it, it is quite clear that water is our most abundant source of fluid and should be the primary drink we intake.

Sugary soft drinks are unfortunately the most common beverage consumed in America today. Not only are these drinks extremely unhealthy but they too are a predominant cause of rising obesity and insulin resistance. Even what many consider to be healthy fruit juices are packed with natural sugar – in any case it is preferable to consume the whole fruit rather than juice it so as to obtain fiber from it.

An alternative to drinking plain water while on the Paleo diet would be tea. Tea (Camellia sinesis) has been drunk for thousands of years in many parts of the world, with its origins being traced to somewhere between modern India and China. This drink is packed with antioxidants which fight off free-radicals that cause ageing and numerous diseases. Drinking tea regularly (especially green and white tea which have the highest levels of antioxidant phytochemicals) can greatly reduce your chances of developing cancer and in many studies have shown to help reverse the effects of cardiovascular disease.

Acid/Alkali Balance

Many of the foods included in the Paleo diet are of an alkaline nature. This is of great value because diets which are considered more acidic have been correlated to high disease incidences such as that of cancer and heart disease. Though there are some acidic foods in the diet (like certain fruits) the overall balance still leans towards the alkaline.

Side effects of Paleo

People commonly complain about feeling lethargic and experiencing headaches and sore muscles after embarking on low-carb diets. Commonly called "carb flu," or keto flu for those on ketogenic diets, the reason for these symptoms remain a mystery.

Metabolically I'm not quite sure what causes it but usually when people have a big change in their diet their body needs some time to adjust.

Generally, you may feel better within a few weeks after starting the diet.

The Paleo Diet, devoid of dairy, also may cause calcium and vitamin D deficiencies

Long-term deficiencies in these two key nutrients could weaken your bones. That said, you can still derive calcium from dark leafy greens and vitamin D from eggs and seafood, both of which you can eat on the Paleo Diet.

Oh, and just so you know, low-carb diets can also lead to constipation, due to the decrease in fiber found in whole grains. Fun!

Is Paleo good for weight loss?

Eating like early man doesn't necessarily mean you'll drop weight. In fact, it's entirely possible you could gain weight on the Paleo Diet.

Yes, some studies indicate that participants on a Paleo diet may have lost weight, but it's not because of anything special within the diet. It's simply because they ate fewer calories overall. Studies have shown that Paleo is ineffective in long-term weight loss. In fact, a study published in JAMA from February 2018 concluded that low-carb diets were not any better than low-fat diets in keeping the weight off.

Is Paleo Gluten Free?

Because a paleo diet excludes all grains - including wheat, rye and barley, a paleo diet is also naturally gluten-free. And for those looking to avoid gluten, paleo options are a safe bet!

How a Paleo Diet Helps With Weight Loss

An added benefit of the paleo diet is the simplicity of it. The rule to "eat foods a caveman would have access to" makes it very easy to shop, plan, and stick with the diet.

Even when eating out, or ordering food, it is still relatively easy to differentiate between processed foods and whole foods "a caveman would have access too."

Because of the simplicity of a paleo diet, it does not require participants to do too much thinking. While calories in versus calories out is the most basic rule to weight loss, a paleo diet takes a lot of thinking out of dieting. As long as you are eating whole, nutritious foods, you will probably find that weight loss will follow naturally—mainly because this style of eating cuts calories automatically.

And while this certainly is not a "one size fits all" approach to dieting, most people will find that if they are filling their body natural, whole, nutrient-dense foods, it will have a substantial impact on your overall weight and body composition as opposed to processed foods.

One study even suggested that your body may burn twice as many calories digesting less processed foods

PALEO DIET VS. KETO:

Which Should I Choose?

If you find yourself asking the paleo diet vs. keto question, you're not alone.

This is one of the most frequently asked questions from those who are new to the paleo diet. Speaking from my own experience, I've found paleo a little easier to follow long-term, though I tend to cycle between keto and paleo (it's the best of both worlds). On both, I maintain a diet that's grain-free, gluten-free and based on whole foods, plenty of veggies and limited dairy. In that respect, both the keto and paleo diets are quite helpful for people like me who have food sensitivities, allergies, and other ingredient intolerances. Of course, it's ultimately about learning which diet works best for you.

I've followed the paleo diet for many years, so I've had plenty of time to explore recipe modifications that keep me feeling happy and satisfied. With dessert recipes like Mexican chocolate mousse and paleo "bread" recipes, I don't even miss my old way of eating at this point. I feel like I can have my (gluten-free) cake and eat it too. And it tastes oh-so-much-sweeter because I feel so much better!

Differences Between Keto And Paleo Diets

The big difference between these two diets is that the keto diet is designed to be a strict, low-carb, high-fat approach to weight loss and dieting. Its goal is to get your body into a state of ketosis. In a nutshell, ketosis shifts your body into a fat reserve-burning mode (versus our more typical carb-burning mode). When you follow a keto diet you'll stick to keto-compliant foods, follow extremely restricted carb intake limits (typically in the ballpark of 20-50 grams per day), and increase your healthy fat intake to help your body adjust to burning fat as fuel.

As far as compliant ingredients go, the biggest differences between the paleo and keto diets are found with dairy, sugars, and fruits. While the paleo diet restricts all dairy ingredients with the single exception of ghee, keto diet followers can have full-fat dairy (like yogurt, heavy cream and cheese). And while the paleo diet allows natural sugars like honey and maple syrup, the keto diet only allows low-carb sweeteners (think ingredients like stevia and monk fruit). Finally, if you're a fruit lover, the keto diet might be challenging – you'll be restricted to low-glycemic fruits like blackberries, raspberries, and strawberries. In comparison, the paleo diet is much less restrictive around your fruit selection.

Similarities Between Paleo And Keto Diets

Of course, there are also similarities between these two diets. There are many foods – and recipes – that overlap and can be enjoyed on both the paleo diet and the keto diet. And both diets avoid foods that are typically higher in carbs like processed foods, fast food, and junk food.

Between these two diets, the paleo diet tends to be the least restrictive. This makes it a great choice if you want to dip your toes into a low carb diet, without needing to track macros. While all the recipes I post on Cook Eat Paleo are paleo-friendly, many are also keto-friendly. And with so many healthy foods that cross over between these two diets, there's no reason why you couldn't mix some keto recipes into your weekly meal plan!

PALEO DIET FOOD LIST

Paleo foods include plenty of plant based fats, grass-fed and wild caught proteins, and nearly all fruits and vegetables. Here are all of the foods considered to be "paleo."

Paleo Proteins

Protein is a staple of the caveman diet- specifically options that are grass-fed, wild caught or organic, as these options are often from animals raised in environments that encourage natural behavior. And because our ancestors didn't just live off chicken and beef, they hunted a wide variety of meat, the more variety you can add to your proteins, the better!

The best paleo proteins include:

Grass-fed Meat

• Beef

• Steak

• Bison

• Pork

• Lamb

• Goat

- Veal

Game Meat

- Venison
- Elk
- Antelope
- Wild Boar
- Rabbit
- Moose
- Emu

Poultry

- Chicken
- Turkey
- Quail
- Goose
- Ostrich
- Duck

Wild Caught Seafood

- Salmon
- Mackerel
- Herring
- Tuna
- Cod
- Tilapia

- Sardines

- Anchovies

- Grouper

- Catfish

- Trout

- Bass

- Haddock

- Walleye

Shellfish

- Shrimp

- Crab

- Clams

- Lobster

- Oysters

- Scallops

- Mussels

- Crawfish

Other Proteins

- Free Range Eggs

Paleo Carbs

Because a paleo diet eliminates all grains, this diet tends to be naturally low in carbohydrates. But if you are looking to add some more carbs to your meal plan, here are the best starchy foods that are also paleo:

Starchy Vegetables

• Sweet Potatoes

• Yams

• Acorn Squash

• Butternut Squash

• Beets

Sugary Fruits

• Mangos

• Apples

• Bananas

• Grapes

• Peaches

• Pears

• Oranges

• Tangerines

• Figs

• Dates

- Guava
- Pineapple
- Papaya
- Lychee

Paleo Fats

Many plant based fats - like nuts and seeds, as well as less processed oils fit into a paleo diet. However, it is important to note that fats are also an easy source of calories and if you are looking to lose weight on a paleo diet, you'll want to limit your portion sizes for these foods:

Nuts and Seeds

- Almonds
- Almond Butter (no added sugar)
- Cashews
- Cashew Butter (no added sugar)
- Hazelnuts
- Pecans
- Walnuts
- Macadamia Nuts
- Chia Seeds
- Flax Seeds

- Sunflower Seeds
- Pine nuts
- Sesame seeds
- Pumpkin seeds

Oils and Butters

- Coconut Oil
- Coconut Butter
- Olive Oil
- Avocado Oil

Other Fats

- Olives
- Avocado
- Tahini
- Shredded Coconut
- Cacao

Paleo Fruits

Just about any fruit or dried fruit (as long as no sugar is added) can fit into your paleo meal plan. Look for more low carb options like these:

- Lemon
- Lime
- Strawberries

• Watermelon

• Raspberries

• Cantaloupe

• Kiwi

• Blackberries

• Plums

• Blueberries

• Jicama

Paleo Veggies

Just like fruit, pretty much all vegetables work on a paleo diet. And non-starchy veggies like the following tend to be low in calories and high in nutrients, meaning your should aim to get a good amount of the following in your diet:

• Kale

• Broccoli Rabe

• Jalapenos

• Watercress

• Bok Choy

• Arugula

• Spinach

• Celery

- Swiss Chard
- Mustard Greens
- Radishes
- Asparagus
- White Mushrooms
- Tomatoes
- Portobello Mushroom
- Onion
- Bamboo Shoots
- Eggplant
- Cucumbers
- Leeks
- Turnips
- Cauliflower
- Bell Peppers
- Kohlrabi
- Broccoli
- Zucchini
- Shiitake Mushrooms
- Okra
- Green Beans (cooked only)
- Cabbage
- Brussel Sprouts

- Carrots

- Fennel

- Oyster Mushrooms

- Rutabaga

- Artichoke

- Pumpkin

Paleo Sweeteners

While majority of added sugar is not paleo friendly, some natural sweeteners can be used in moderation on this diet:

Natural sweeteners

- Honey

- Maple Syrup

- Coconut Sugar

- Date Paste

Paleo Drinks

Look for simple drink options, made without artificial sweetener or too much added sugar, like the following:

- Water

- Coffee (No cream or sugar)

- Unsweetened Teas
- Coconut water
- Bone broth
- Sparkling Water (no added sugar or artificial sweetener)

Non-Paleo Foods To Avoid

While a paleo diet has a general "whole food" approach to eating, there are still many traditional health foods that are not considered paleo - like dairy, legumes and whole grains, because they were not commonly consumed by our ancestors.

A more controversial argument for why legumes and common grains are avoided is because of their high phytic acid content, which is thought to reduce the absorption of certain nutrients like iron zinc and calcium. However, phytic acid is also found in many paleo approved foods (like almonds and hazelnuts), and is associated with some health benefits - like protective benefits against kidney stones, antioxidant properties and a suggested link to lower risk for colon cancer. Bottom line, there really isn't any evidenced based reason to avoid these foods because of phytic acid.

And as for dairy, the research behind whether or not dairy is bad for you, isn't very conclusive either.

Some people have digestive issues when eating beans, legumes, grains anddairy, for a variety of health reasons. And if any of these foods don't work with your body, this is probably the best excuses to avoid them.

Because of the debate around these foods, there is a lot of confusion, and some people will choose a more modified paleo diet that still has some dairy or legumes included. But a true paleo diet does not include any of the following:

Beans and Legumes

• Beans

• Lentils

• Green Peas

• Chickpeas

• Snow Peas

• Soy Beans

• Tofu

• Miso

- Peanuts

- Peanut Butter

Dairy

- Cows Milk

- Goats Milk

- Sheep's Milk

- Cheese

- Cottage Cheese

- Cream

- Butter

- Ice cream

- Yogurt

Grains

- Quinoa

- Rice

- Oats

- Wheat

- Corn

- Pasta

- Bread

- Crackers

- Barley
- Ancient Grains
- Cereal Grains

Starchy Veggies

- Regular Potatoes
- Yucca

Processed Cooking Oils

- Vegetable Oil
- Canola Oil
- Corn Oil
- Peanut Oil
- Palm Oil

Other Processed Foods and Ingredients

- Artificial Sweeteners: Aspartame, neotame, saccharin, sucralose, xylitol, erythritol
- Refined Sugars: Brown sugar, table sugar, agave, corn syrup
- Processed Meats: hot dogs, spam
- Packaged Foods and Snacks
- Fruit Juices

- Candy

- Chips

- Popcorn

- Soda

- Alcohol

Tips For Shopping Paleo

If you are new to eating paleo, this may seem like a big change to your life. Cutting out grains, processed foods, dairy, and a load of other relatively common items may seem overwhelming.

Here are some tips we have to simplify the process and put your worries at ease.

1) Plan Your Meals

If you are struggling on where to begin, planning out meals that you enjoy and then figuring out a way to make that meal paleo will be a good place to start. Instead of immediately switching to a diet full of chicken and broccoli, find ways to get creative with the process so that you can cook food you genuinely enjoy.

Yes, even paleo food can be delicious; it just takes a little bit of creativity and stepping outside of your comfort zone. Here are some ideas for creative paleo meals.

2) Make A List

Once you have decided what meals you want to make for the week, create a list of all of the ingredients you need to make that food. As simple as this sounds, it will make it much easier for you to stick to a set plan and not get too deep into the aisles of a grocery store. Having something as simple as a grocery list will keep you on track and ensure you get exactly what you came for. It will also help familiarize you with where to find these paleo-friendly foods in your local store.

3) Shop Outside The Aisles

If all else fails, this simple rule of thumb may make it really easy to shop for paleo foods. The layout of most grocery stores is quite simple: in the inner aislesyou will typically find packaged, processed foods. Things like bread, pasta, cereal, flour, sugar, etc. For the most part, many of the foods stocked in the inner aisles of a grocery store will probably be "non-paleo approved items."

Every now and then you may find some "paleo" food items in the inner aisles (a lot of paleo-approved flours may be in the inner aisles of a grocery store), but that is an exception, not the rule.

Typically, if you are shopping the outer aisles of a grocery store there will be a produce, meat, poultry, eggs, and bulk food section. All of these areas tend to provide you with the foundation of a paleo diet, including fruits, vegetables, nuts, and meats.

If you find yourself lacking a clear direction when grocery shopping, using this simple rule should help you create a clear path and help you avoid the variety of temptation within the aisles.

TIPS TO GETTING STARTED

Of course, it's always a good idea to check in with your doctor whenever you decide to change your diet. It will help you understand any current restrictions for your health. And help you establish a baseline, so you can see how a healthier diet based on eating whole foods actually helps you improve your health over time.

Ready to get started? Here are the top tips I recommend for those new to paleo:

1. BEGIN WITH EASY PALEO RECIPES

The best way to start is to just try making a paleo meal. Simple, right? Choose a couple of easy recipes, pick up your paleo ingredients, and give those healthy recipes a spin. And with kitchen gadgets like the Instant Pot and slow cooker, easy paleo recipes are even easier. Even if you're really busy and completely strapped for time. Even on incredibly busy weeknights! If you can carve out even 5 minutes of hands-on prep time, you have enough time to make a quick paleo recipe (like this Instant Pot salsa chicken).

2. MEAL PREP YOUR PALEO MEALS

Another easy way to get started is to cook your meals in advance. If you're really struggling to find time during the week, try setting aside an hour or two on the weekend to meal prep some of your paleo ingredients for the week ahead. You'll often find me prepping a whole chicken (this is the easiest "roast" chicken recipe!) for shredding in my lunches. And it only takes 10 minutes to batch prepare this freezer-friendly cauliflower rice. Soups, stews and even muffins are other perfect candidates for meal prepping in advance. Just throw them in the freezer until you're ready to serve them!

3. CHOOSE PALEO RECIPES YOU ACTUALLY LIKE

Of course, an important part of being able to stick with the paleo diet is actually enjoying the food you're eating. Try looking for healthier versions of your favorite recipes. Whether that's pulled pork sandwiches or café-worthy banana bread, it really doesn't matter. The key is finding recipes that you love and feel great serving. It's not so hard to stay on track when you can't wait to cook up your favorite dishes!

4. MEAL PLAN FOR (PALEO) SUCCESS

Once you start to gather recipes that you love, you'll begin to build meal plans that support your new healthy eating goals. Meal planning can sometimes feel overwhelming, but it can also free you from stressing about what's for dinner. Armed with meal planning best practices (like planning to plan!) will help keep this activity easy and stress-free.

SIMPLE PALEO RECIPES TO KICKSTART YOUR MEAL PLAN

Once you get to the point that you're actively building your paleo meal plan, you'll want to start gathering paleo recipes to refer back to during planning sessions. With these handy paleo recipe collections on hand, you'll be ready to breeze through planning your paleo meal plan.

BREAKFAST IDEAS

Quick and easy breakfasts are one of the biggest challenges when you first go paleo. Luckily, with these fast paleo breakfast ideas will make mornings a breeze. You'll be covered no matter whether you choose a smoothie, granola or meal prep some freezer-friendly breakfast sausages.

Cranberry Walnut Paleo Granola

This quick and easy grain-free cranberry walnut granola is crunchy and naturally sweet.

Prep Time: 5 mins

Cook Time: 20 mins

Total Time: 25 mins

Servings: 24 1/4-cup servings (6 cups)

Calories: 163kcal

Ingredients

• 2 cups chopped walnuts

• 1 cup slivered almonds

• 1 cup raw pepitas or pumpkin seeds

• 1 cup unsweetened shredded coconut

• 1/4 teaspoon sea salt

• 2 tablespoons coconut oil melted

• 3 tablespoons honey or maple syrup

• 1 cup dried cranberries apple juice sweetened

Instructions

1. Preheat oven to 300 degrees.

2. Combine nuts, seeds, coconut and salt in large bowl.

3. Add coconut oil and honey and mix until well combined.

4. Bake on a rimmed cookie sheet lined with parchment paper (or prepared with cooking spray) for 18 - 20 minutes, until just lightly browned.

5. Add the dried cranberries and toss to combine. Cool completely before serving.

Nutrition

Calories: 163kcal | Carbohydrates: 9g | Protein: 3g | Fat: 13g | Saturated Fat: 4g | Cholesterol: 0mg | Sodium: 26mg | Potassium: 119mg | Fiber: 2g | Sugar: 6g | Vitamin C: 0.2mg | Calcium: 24mg | Iron: 0.8mg

Paleo Breakfast Sausage

This quick and easy paleo breakfast sausage has just a few ingredients, and comes together in minutes.

Prep Time: 10 mins

Cook Time: 10 mins

Total Time: 20 mins

Servings: 8 patties

Calories: 150kcal

Ingredients

• 1 pound ground pork

• 1 teaspoon rubbed sage

• 1/2 teaspoon smoked sweet paprika

• 1/2 teaspoon smoked hot paprika

• 1 teaspoon sea salt

• 3/4 teaspoon fresh ground pepper

Instructions

1. Combine spices in small bowl. Add to ground pork and mix until just combined. Form into 8 patties.

2. Cook patties in a skillet over medium-low heat until browned and cooked through.

Nutrition

Calories: 150kcal | Carbohydrates: 0g | Protein: 9g | Fat: 12g | Saturated Fat: 4g | Cholesterol: 40mg |

Sodium: 322mg | Potassium: 162mg | Fiber: 0g | Sugar: 0g | Vitamin A: 125IU | Vitamin C: 0.4mg | Calcium: 8mg | Iron: 0.6mg

Paleo Blueberry Muffin Recipe

These gluten-free blueberry muffins are a delicious way to start the day.

Prep Time: 10 mins

Cook Time: 25 mins

Total Time: 35 mins

Servings: 9 muffins

Calories: 215kcal

Ingredients

• 200 grams fine almond flour about 2 cups

• 1/2 teaspoon baking soda

• 1/8 teaspoon fine sea salt

• 3 eggs

• 1/4 cup honey

• 2 tablespoons ghee or coconut oil, melted

• 1 tablespoon lemon juice

• 1 teaspoon organic vanilla extract

• 1 cup fresh blueberries

Instructions

1. Preheat oven to 325 degrees and grease or line muffin tin.

2. Combine dry Ingredientsin large bowl. Combine wet Ingredientsin medium bowl. Stir wet ingredients into dry ingredients, then fold in blueberries.

3. Using a large scoop, fill muffin cups 3/4 full.

4. Bake for 20 - 25 minutes, until golden brown and toothpick inserted in center comes out clean. Cool on wire rack.

Nutrition

Calories: 215kcal | Carbohydrates: 15g | Protein: 6g | Fat: 15g | Saturated Fat: 3g | Cholesterol: 63mg | Sodium: 114mg | Potassium: 37mg | Fiber: 2g | Sugar: 10g | Vitamin A: 90IU | Vitamin C: 2.2mg | Calcium: 55mg | Iron: 1.2mg

Espresso Protein Shake

This espresso protein shake is creamy and thick like a frozen coffee shop drink.

Prep Time: 5 mins

Total Time: 5 mins

Servings: 1 serving

Ingredients

- 1/2 cup cashew milk

- 1/2 banana frozen

- 2/3 cup ice cubes

- 1/2 teaspoon vanilla extract

- dash of cinnamon

- 1/4 cup unflavored egg white protein powder

- 2 ounces espresso or strong coffee

- honey or sweetener of choice optional

Instructions

1. Add all Ingredientsto Vitamix and blend on high until smooth. Pour into a tall glass and serve.

Sausage and Butternut Squash Frittata

This quick and easy sausage and squash frittata is perfect for breakfast, lunch or dinner.

Prep Time: 5 mins

Cook Time: 15 mins

Total Time: 20 mins

Servings: 2 servings

Calories: 341kcal

Ingredients

• 1 tablespoon bacon fat duck fat or fat of choice

• 3 ounces cooked sausage chopped or crumbled

• 1/4 cup onion diced

• 1/4 cup red pepper diced

• 1/2 cup butternut squash cubed and roasted

• 3 large eggs

• 2 teaspoons mixed fresh herbs or 1/2 teaspoon dried

• sea salt and pepper to taste

Instructions

1. Preheat broiler.

2. Beat eggs, salt and pepper and herbs until well-combined.

3. Add fat to 10-inch oven-proof skillet and sauté onions and peppers until soft. Add sausage and

squash and cook until heated through. Pour eggs over filling and cook until edges start to set.

4. Put pan in oven and broil until frittata is puffed and brown on top, 3-5 minutes.

Nutrition

Calories: 341kcal | Carbohydrates: 8g | Protein: 16g | Fat: 26g | Saturated Fat: 8g | Cholesterol: 282mg | Sodium: 378mg | Potassium: 424mg | Fiber: 2g | Sugar: 2g | Vitamin A: 4690IU | Vitamin C: 32.6mg| Calcium: 67mg | Iron: 2.3mg

Cranberry Orange Scones

A perfect not-too-sweet treat for breakfast or an afternoon snack.

Prep Time: 10 mins

Cook Time: 20 mins

Total Time: 30 mins

Servings: 9 scones

Calories: 247kcal

Ingredients

• 315 grams almond flour about 3 cups

• 1 teaspoon baking soda

• ⅛ teaspoon fine sea salt

- 1 teaspoon orange zest

- ½ cup dried cranberries apple juice sweetened

- 2 eggs

- 2 tablespoons honey

- ⅛ teaspoon orange extract

- 1 tablespoon fresh lemon juice or fresh-squeezed orange juice

Instructions

1. Preheat oven to 325 degrees.

2. Add the almond flour, baking soda, salt, orange zest and cranberries to a large bowl and stir to combine.

3. Make a well in the center of the flour mixture and add the remaining ingredients. Starting in the center, stir the dough until well combined.

4. Using a large cookie or ice cream scoop, drop the scones onto a baking sheet lined with parchment paper. Lightly wet hands and gently flatten the tops of the scones. They should be about 1 inch thick.

5. Bake 18-20 minutes, until the tops are golden brown. Cool on wire rack.

Calories: 247kcal | Carbohydrates: 17g | Protein: 9g | Fat: 18g | Saturated Fat: 2g | Cholesterol: 36mg | Sodium: 168mg | Potassium: 13mg | Fiber: 4g | Sugar: 10g | Vitamin A: 53IU | Vitamin C: 1mg | Calcium: 79mg | Iron: 2mg

Paleo "Instant Oatmeal" Recipe

An easy gluten-free hot breakfast to take the place of regular instant oatmeal.

Prep Time: 3 mins

Cook Time: 2 mins

Total Time: 5 mins

Servings: 1 serving

Calories: 231kcal

Ingredients

• 1/2 banana

• 2 tablespoons unsweetened shredded coconut

• 2 tablespoons almond flour

• 1/3 - 1/2 cup cashew milk

• 1/4 teaspoon cinnamon

• pinch of sea salt

Instructions

1. Mash banana in bottom of bowl. Add remaining Ingredientsand stir to combine.

2. Microwave 1 - 2 minutes, until hot and starting to bubble. Stir and let stand a couple minutes. It will thicken slightly as it cools.

3. Serve with your favorite toppings.

Nutrition

Calories: 231kcal | Carbohydrates: 20g | Protein: 4g | Fat: 16g | Saturated Fat: 9g | Cholesterol: 0mg | Sodium: 6mg | Potassium: 292mg | Fiber: 5g | Sugar: 8g | Vitamin C: 5.1mg | Calcium: 29mg | Iron: 1mg

HEALTHY PALEO LUNCH IDEAS

Of course, your paleo meal plan wouldn't be complete without healthy paleo lunch recipes. Each of these paleo lunch recipes is loaded with fresh ingredients, protein and plenty of healthy fats. Perfect for keeping you energized and full until it's time for dinner!

Avocado Tuna Salad (Paleo, Keto, Whole30)
An easy no-mayo quick and easy healthy snack or lunch.
Prep Time: 5 mins
Total Time: 5 mins
Servings: 2 servings
Calories: 239kcal
Ingredients
• 1 avocado
• 1 lemon juiced, to taste
• 1 tablespoon chopped onion to taste
• 5 ounces cooked or canned wild tuna
• sea salt to taste
• fresh ground pepper to taste

Instructions

1. Cut the avocado in half and scoop the middle of both avocado halves into a bowl, leaving a shell of avocado flesh about 1/4-inch thick on each half.

2. Add lemon juice and onion to the avocado in the bowl and mash together. Add tuna, salt and pepper, and stir to combine. Taste and adjust if needed.

3. Fill avocado shells with tuna salad and serve.

Nutrition

Calories: 239kcal | Carbohydrates: 14g | Protein: 16g | Fat: 15g | Saturated Fat: 2g | Cholesterol: 25mg | Sodium: 183mg | Potassium: 688mg | Fiber: 8g | Sugar: 2g | Vitamin A: 185IU | Vitamin C: 38.7mg | Calcium: 38mg | Iron: 2mg

The No Bread BLT

Yield: 1 Serving

Prep Time: 10 Minutes

Cook Time: 10 Minutes

Total Time: 20 Minutes

Ingredients

• 6 slices bacon, cut in half horizontally

• lettuce leaves

• fresh tomato, sliced

Instructions

1. Place three slices next to each other in a vertical row on a baking tray lined with a silicone mat.

2. Flap the top of the outer two slices down, then place a slice of bacon horizontally across them.

3. Flap the bacon back up, then flap up the central slice, and place another horizontal slice in the middle. Then add the final horizontal slice at the bottom by flapping up the two outer slices.

4. Repeat to form another bacon weave (you will need two per BLT).

5. Place an inverted non-stick rack over the top of the bacon and cook under a preheated broiler until the bacon starts to go crispy. Remove the rack, and flip over the bacon. Return to the broiler if necessary.

6. Transfer the bacon weaves to kitchen paper to drain the excess fat.

7. Add sliced tomato and crunchy romaine lettuce to one bacon weave, then top with the second weave.

Nutrition Information

Calories: 563 | Total Fat: 52g | Saturated Fat: 17g |
Cholesterol: 87mg | Sodium: 883mg | Carbohydrates:

4g | Net Carbohydrates: 4g | Fiber: 0g | Sugar: 1g | Protein| 17g

Raw Vegetable Nori Rolls Or Wraps With Sunflower Seed Butter Dipping Sauce (Raw, Vegan, Grain-Free, Paleo)

Yields: Makes 6 To 8 Wraps

Raw vegetables are bundled up in a nori sheet and served alongside a creamy sunflower butter dip.

Prep Time: 25 min

Ingredients

To make the sunflower seed dipping sauce:

• 1/4 Cup/60g sunflower seed butter (or use a raw sunflower seed butter for an entirely raw sauce)

• 1 Tablespoon/15ml coconut aminos

• 1 Tablespoon/15ml freshly squeezed lime juice

• 1 teaspoon/5ml sesame oil (or use untoasted to keep the recipe entirely raw)

• 1 teaspoon/5ml maple syrup

• 1/8 tsp red pepper flakes

• Hot water to thin

To make the carrot "rice":

• 4 medium carrots, peeled, roughly chopped

• 1 teaspoon/5ml raw apple cider vinegar or raw coconut vinegar

To make the vegetable nori rolls:

• 3 to 4 Nori sheets

• 1 recipe for carrot "rice" (see above)

• 1 medium watermelon radish, julienned

• ½ a large avocado, thinly sliced (optional)

• 1 cup baby spinach leaves

• 1 cup sprouts of your choice such as sunflower or pea

Instructions

Make the sunflower seed butter sauce:

1. Whisk all the Ingredientstogether adding enough hot water to thin to make a loose but not watery sauce for dipping.

Make the carrot "rice":

2. Pulse the carrots in the bowl of a food processor until very finely chopped (about the size of rice).

3. Remove the chopped carrots and place in the middle of a clean kitchen towel, cheesecloth or nut bag squeezing over a large bowl to remove the liquid. Save the juice and drink it, you just made carrot juice without a juicer! (Alternatively you can use the leftover

carrot pulp from making carrot juice to make the carrot rice.)

4. Place the carrot "rice" in bowl and add vinegar, stir to combine.

5. Place a nori sheet shiny side down on a sushi mat or cutting board. Spoon a thin layer of the carrot "rice" along a third of the sheet closest to you, pressing down firmly to smooth.

6. Place the spinach in the middle of the carrot "rice" all the way down the sheet. Repeat with the avocado, radishes and sprouts.

7. Using the edge of the sushi mat closest to you, grasp the mat and the edge of the nori sheet rolling both over the vegetable filling. Press down on the opposite side pulling back gently towards you to create a log shape. Roll nori tightly, using the mat to help. Brush the edge of the nori sheet furthest away from you with a finger dipped in a little water to moisten and seal the edge.

8. Repeat this process until you have run out of filling or nori sheets.

9. Place the rolls seam side down and using a sharp knife, gently slice the nori rolls into desired pieces and arrange on a serving platter . Serve the rolls immediately with the dipping sauce alongside.

Bacon Wrapped Apple Pork Meatball Kebabs

Servings: 6 kebabs

Ingredients

- 450 g pastured ground pork
- 1 small onion, finely chopped
- ½ red cooking apple, finely chopped
- 1 tsp salt
- 1 tsp black pepper
- 1 tsp chai spice
- ¼ cup fresh parsley, finely chopped
- ¼ cup fresh mint, finely chopped
- ¼ cup raisins
- 1 egg, lightly beaten
- ¼ cup coconut flour
- 9 slices pastured bacon, cut in half
- 1 red cooking apple, peel on, cored and cut into 8 wedges
- 6 wooden or metal kebab skewers

Instructions

1. If using wooden skewers, put them in cold water to soak for at least 30 minutes prior to using them.

2. Place all the ingredients except for bacon and apple wedges in a large mixing bowl and knead well with your hands until uniformly blended. Form the meat mixture into 18 medium sized meatballs.

3. Wrap half a bacon slice around each meatball, making sure that it wraps completely around the meatballs and even overlaps a little bit. If necessary, don't hesitate to reshape your meatballs and make them slightly oval.

4. Cut each apple wedge in half crosswise.

5. Thread 3 meatballs and 2 pieces of apple per skewer, alternating between meat and fruit. When threading the meatballs, make sure that you insert the skewer right through that spot where the bacon overlaps. This will prevent the bacon from coming undone on the grill.

6. Preheat your grill to medium-high heat.

7. Place the kabobs on the grill and cook until the meatballs are cooked through and the bacon is nice and crispy, about 3-4 minutes per side.

8. Serve immediately with loads of fresh veggies.

5-minute turkey cranberry lettuce wraps

Fast, simple, and ultra flavorful, 15-Minute Turkey Cranberry Lettuce Wraps make a delicious weeknight meal and come together in just minutes.

Ingredients

• 2 tablespoons olive oil, divided

• 1 medium yellow onion, finely chopped

• ½ teaspoon salt, divided

• 2 garlic cloves, finely minced or grated

• 1 pound ground dark or light meat turkey

• ¼ cup dried, unsweetened or apple juice sweetened cranberries*

• Juice of half a lime (about 1 tablespoon)

• 2 tablespoons chopped fresh sage

• 1 head butter lettuce or radicchio

Instructions

1. In a large pan, heat 1 tablespoon olive oil over medium heat. Add the onion, sprinkle with ¼ teaspoon salt, and sauté, stirring frequently, until translucent and cooked through, about 5-8 minutes.

2. Add an additional 1 tablespoon olive oil, garlic, and turkey. Sprinkle with an additional ¼ teaspoon salt, then sauté, stirring occasionally, until the turkey is browned and cooked through, about 5 minutes.

3. Add the cranberries, lime juice, and sage, stirring to combine.

4. Serve warm, wrapped in lettuce cups.

Salmon Lettuce Wraps with Cucumber, Jicama, and Ginger Recipe

• Prep time: 30 minutes

• Cook time: 20 minutes

• Yield: Serves 4

Prep the Ingredientsfor the cucumber, jicama, ginger salad while the salmon fillets are marinating.

Ingredients

• 12 ounces skinless salmon fillets, cut into two even pieces

• 1/2 teaspoon Kosher salt for marinade

• 1 teaspoon grated fresh ginger root

• 4 cups water

• 1 1/2 teaspoons Kosher salt for poaching liquid

• Slice of lemon

- 1 teaspoon extra virgin olive oil
- 1 teaspoon lemon juice

Cucumber, Jicama, Ginger Salad:

- 3/4 cup of seeded, diced, thin-skinned (English or Persian) cucumber, peel-on (you can also use regular cucumbers that have been peeled)
- 2/3 cup peeled, small diced jicama
- 1/4 thinly sliced red onion
- 3 Tbsp chopped fresh cilantro
- 1 teaspoon grated lime zest
- 2 Tbsp fresh lime juice
- 2 teaspoons grated fresh ginger
- 1 Tbsp chopped fresh mint
- 1/2 teaspoon Kosher salt
- 1 ripe avocado
- 6 large leaves of butter lettuce

Instructions

1 Marinate the salmon fillets: Rub with 1/2 teaspoon Kosher salt and a teaspoon of grated ginger. Set in refrigerator to chill for 30 minutes, while you prep the other ingredients.

2 Combine cucumbers, jicama, red onion, cilantro, lime, ginger, mint, salt: In a medium bowl, gently

combine the diced cucumbers, jicama, red onion, cilantro, lime zest, lime juice, grated ginger, chopped mint, and salt. Set aside for the flavors to blend.

3 Poach the salmon: Prepare salmon poaching liquid. Place water, salt, and a slice of lemon in a pot wide enough to hold the salmon fillets. Bring to a boil and let simmer for about 5 minutes.

Add the salmon fillets that have been marinating in ginger and salt to the poaching liquid. Return to a simmer and cook for about 4 minute at a very low simmer.

When just cooked through, remove from poaching liquid and place in a bowl. Toss with a teaspoon of olive oil and a teaspoon of lemon juice. Once the salmon has cooled to touch, break up gently into large flakes.

4 Arrange the lettuce wraps: Slice the avocado. On to each butter lettuce leaf, place a few chunks of salmon, a large spoonful of the cucumber jicama mixture, and top with some slices of avocado.

Fold up the lettuce wrap and eat!

Power Greens Salad With Blueberries

Power Greens Salad with Blueberries will help you eat your SuperFoods, this healthy salad is also delicious!

Yield: 2 Servings

Prep Time: 15 Minutes

Total Time: 15 Minutes

INGREDIENTS:

• 5 oz. Power Greens mix of baby kale, spinach, and chard (or any mix of greens of your choice)

• 1 cup fresh blueberries

• 1/4 cup slivered almonds, toasted

DRESSING INGREDIENTS:

• 1 large lemon (zested and squeezed to get 1 tsp. lemon zest and 2 T lemon juice)

• 3 T extra-virgin olive oil

• 1/4 tsp. mustard (choose mustard without added sugar for Whole 30/Paleo diet)

• salt and fresh-ground black pepper to taste

INSTRUCTIONS

1. Put greens in a salad spinner and soak in very cold water for 5 minutes to crisp the greens. (If your greens are really fresh, they may not need this.)

2. While greens soak, measure 1 cup blueberries, picking them over to remove any soft ones.

3. Zest the lemon and then squeeze the juice to get 1 tsp. zest and 2 T juice; then whisk together the lemon zest, lemon juice, olive oil, mustard, salt, and pepper to make the dressing.

4. Toast the almonds in a dry pan over high heat until they barely start to get some color (only a minute or so.)

5. Spin the greens until they're very dry or pat dry with paper towels.

6. Put greens into a salad bowl and toss with desired amount of dressing, until the greens are as moist as you prefer.

7. Divide greens between two salad bowls and toss each with half the blueberries and half the almonds.

8. Serve right away.

Chicken Salad with Grapes and Walnuts

An easy and healthy version of the restaurant classic chicken salad with grapes.

Prep Time: 10 mins

Total Time10 mins

Servings: 4 servings

Calories: 405kcal

Ingredients

• 2 tablespoons minced shallot

• 2 tablespoons fresh lemon juice

• 1/4 cup extra virgin olive oil

• salt and fresh ground pepper

• 2 cups diced cooked organic chicken

• 1 cup halved organic seedless grapes

• 1/2 cup chopped walnuts

• 1/2 cup diced organic celery

• 2 tablespoons fresh chopped parsley

Instructions

1. Add shallots and lemon juice to medium bowl. Whisk in olive oil slowly until dressing is emulsified. Season with salt and pepper to taste.

2. Add chicken, grapes, walnuts, celery, and parsley to bowl with dressing. Toss to combine. Taste and adjust seasonings.

Nutrition

Calories: 405kcal | Carbohydrates: 10g | Protein: 19g | Fat: 32g | Saturated Fat: 5g | Cholesterol: 53mg | Sodium: 64mg | Potassium: 344mg | Fiber: 1g | Sugar:

7g | Vitamin A: 310IU | Vitamin C: 7.6mg | Calcium: 34mg | Iron: 1.7mg

Paleo burrito bowl recipe (21dsd)

Prep Time: 10 Mins

Cook Time: 10 Mins

Total Time: 20 Mins

Yield: 4 servings

Ingredients

• 2 tablespoons coconut oil

• 1 large onion, chopped

• 1 cup sliced black olives

• 3 cups riced cauliflower

• 2 cups leftover taco-spiced beef

• 4 roma tomatoes, chopped

• 5 cups shredded lettuce

• 1 ripe avocado, sliced

• 1 cup salsa

• Diced cilantro

Instructions

1. Saute the onion, olives, and cauliflower in coconut oil until soft. Add the the taco meat and tomatoes and

cook until hot. Serve over shredded lettuce and top with salsa, sliced avocado, and diced cilantro! Boom!

Serving Size: 1/4 of recipe | Calories: 515 | Fat: 28.2g | Saturated fat: 11.2 g | Unsaturated fat: 7g | Trans fat: 0g | Carbohydrates: 27.9g | Sugar: 10.2g | Sodium: 1167mg | Fiber: 10.8g | Protein: 40.8g | Cholesterol: 101mg

EASY PALEO SNACKS

These quick, easy paleo snack recipes are the perfect choice if you're planning for a mid-afternoon treat. Whether you're in the mood for some paleo snack mix, a gluten-free muffin, some deviled eggs, or a dip served with crunchy veggies, these easy snack ideas are a perfect choice.

Paleo Snack Mix Recipe

This paleo snack mix is salty, smoky and garlicky, just like traditional bar snacks.

Prep Time: 5 mins

Cook Time: 20 mins

Total Time: 25 mins

Servings: 12 servings (3 cups)

Calories: 184kcal

Ingredients

- 1 cup sliced almonds
- 1 cup walnuts
- 1 cup pecans
- 1 tablespoon garlic infused olive oil
- 1-2 teaspoons smoked sea salt to taste

• 1 teaspoon smoked sweet paprika

• 1/4 - 1/2 teaspoon smoked hot paprika to taste

Instructions

1. Preheat oven to 325 degrees.

2. Combine nuts in a large bowl and toss with olive oil until well coated.

3. Combine salt and spices in a small bowl. Sprinkle over nuts and stir until well combined.

4. Spread nuts in single layer on baking sheet. Bake 15-20 minutes or until lightly browned and crispy.

Nutrition

Calories: 184kcal | Carbohydrates: 4g | Protein: 4g | Fat: 18g | Saturated Fat: 1g | Cholesterol: 0mg | Sodium: 195mg | Potassium: 139mg | Fiber: 2g | Sugar: 1g | Vitamin A: 85IU | Vitamin C: 0.2mg | Calcium: 37mg | Iron: 0.8mg

Avocado Tuna Salad (Paleo, Keto, Whole30)

An easy no-mayo quick and easy healthy snack or lunch.

Prep Time: 5 mins

Total Time5 mins

Servings: 2 servings

Calories: 239kcal

Ingredients

• 1 avocado

• 1 lemon juiced, to taste

• 1 tablespoon chopped onion to taste

• 5 ounces cooked or canned wild tuna

• sea salt to taste

• fresh ground pepper to taste

Instructions

1. Cut the avocado in half and scoop the middle of both avocado halves into a bowl, leaving a shell of avocado flesh about 1/4-inch thick on each half.

2. Add lemon juice and onion to the avocado in the bowl and mash together. Add tuna, salt and pepper, and stir to combine. Taste and adjust if needed.

3. Fill avocado shells with tuna salad and serve.

Nutrition

Calories: 239kcal | Carbohydrates: 14g | Protein: 16g | Fat: 15g | Saturated Fat: 2g | Cholesterol: 25mg | Sodium: 183mg | Potassium: 688mg | Fiber: 8g | Sugar: 2g | Vitamin A: 185IU | Vitamin C: 38.7mg | Calcium: 38mg | Iron: 2mg

Lemon Poppy Paleo Muffins

Prep Time: 5 mins

Cook Time: 25 mins

Total Time: 30 mins

Servings: 8 muffins

Calories: 143kcal

Ingredients

• 4 eggs

• zest of one lemon

• 3 tablespoons lemon juice

• 1/4 cup ghee melted (can substitute coconut oil)

• 1/4 cup honey

• 1 teaspoon vanilla extract

• 1/8 teaspoon salt

• 1/3 cup coconut flour

• 1/2 teaspoon baking soda

• 1 tablespoon poppy seeds

Instructions

1. Preheat oven to 350 degrees. Grease or line muffin tin.

2. Add all ingredients except poppy seeds to food processor and process until well combined. Pulse in poppy seeds.

3. Bake 25-30 minutes until golden brown and toothpick inserted in center comes out clean. Cool completely on wire rack.

Nutrition

Calories: 143kcal | Carbohydrates: 12g | Protein: 3g | Fat: 8g | Saturated Fat: 4g | Cholesterol: 96mg | Sodium: 147mg | Potassium: 49mg | Fiber: 2g | Sugar: 9g | Vitamin A: 120IU | Vitamin C: 3.1mg | Calcium: 28mg | Iron: 0.7mg

Deviled Eggs with Bacon and Chives

Deviled eggs are a quick snack or easy appetizer. This simple recipe is a perfect base for bacon, chives, roasted red peppers, and olives.

Prep Time: 15 mins

Total Time15 mins

Servings: 6 servings

Calories: 131kcal

Ingredients

• 6 hard-boiled eggs

• 1 tablespoon whole grain Dijon mustard

• 1 tablespoon olive oil

• 1 teaspoon garlic infused olive oil

• 1 - 2 teaspoons lemon juice

• sea salt & pepper to taste

Toppings

• 2 tablespoons crumbled cooked bacon

• 2 tablespoons snipped chives

• 2 tablespoons sliced olives

• 2 tablespoons chopped roasted red peppers

Instructions

1. Peel eggs and slice in half lengthwise. Place egg whites on serving tray and add egg yolks to mixing bowl.

2. Add mustard, olive oils, lemon juice, salt and pepper to egg yolks. Mash with fork until creamy. If needed, add water to thin, one teaspoon at a time. Taste and adjust seasonings.

3. Fill egg whites with yolk mixture and top generously with desired toppings.

Nutrition

Calories: 131kcal | Carbohydrates: 1g | Protein: 7g | Fat: 10g | Saturated Fat: 2g | Cholesterol: 189mg | Sodium: 232mg | Potassium: 79mg | Fiber: 0g | Sugar: 0g | Vitamin A: 340IU | Vitamin C: 3.4mg | Calcium: 27mg | Iron: 0.7mg

Paleo Ranch Dressing and Dip

Prep Time: 5 mins

Total Time5 mins

Servings: 20 servings (makes 1-1/4 cups)

Calories: 82kcal

Ingredients

• 1 cup paleo mayonnaise

• 2 tablespoons lemon juice

• 1/4 cup full fat coconut milk

• 1 clove garlic minced

• 2 tablespoons minced fresh herbs parsley, basil and chives

• sea salt and freshly cracked black pepper to taste

Instructions

1. Whisk all ingredients together.

2. Taste and adjust seasonings.

Nutrition

Serving: 1tablespoon | Calories: 82kcal | Carbohydrates: 0g | Protein: 0g | Fat: 8g | Saturated Fat: 1g | Cholesterol: 4mg | Sodium: 71mg | Potassium: 10mg | Fiber: 0g | Sugar: 0g | Vitamin A: 40IU | Vitamin C: 1.2mg | Calcium: 2mg | Iron: 0.1mg

Blueberry Pecan Paleo Granola

Servings: 3 cups

Ingredients

• 1 cup chopped pecans

• 1 cup sliced almonds

• 1/2 cup sunflower seeds

• 1/2 cup finely shredded unsweetened coconut

• 1/4 teaspoon sea salt

• 1 tablespoon grass-fed ghee or coconut oil melted

• 3 tablespoons pure maple syrup

• 1/2 cup organic dried blueberries

Instructions

1. Preheat oven to 325 degrees.

2. Combine pecans, almonds, sunflower seeds, coconut and salt in large bowl.

3. Combine ghee or coconut oil with maple syrup. Stir into nut mixture until well combined.

4. Bake on a rimmed baking sheet lined with parchment paper for 12 - 15 minutes, until just lightly browned.

5. Add the dried blueberries and toss to combine. Cool completely before serving.

Roasted Cauliflower Hummus

This cauliflower hummus recipe is a perfect blend of tahini, lemon, and garlic.

Prep Time: 15 mins

Cook Time: 20 mins

Servings: 6 servings

Calories: 211kcal

Ingredients

- 1 head cauliflower cut into florets
- 1/3 cup extra virgin olive oil divided
- 1/3 cup tahini
- 1 clove garlic peeled
- juice of 2 lemons
- 1/2 - 1 teaspoon sea salt to taste

Instructions

1. Preheat oven to 425 degrees.

2. Toss cauliflower florets with 1 tablespoon olive oil and a pinch of salt. Roast on a rimmed baking sheet until fork tender and caramelized, about 20 minutes. Cool completely.

3. Add roasted cauliflower, tahini, garlic, lemon juice, salt, and olive oil to food processor. Process until

mixture reaches hummus consistency. Taste and adjust seasonings. Add water, if needed, to thin.

Nutrition

Calories: 211kcal | Carbohydrates: 8g | Protein: 4g | Fat: 19g | Saturated Fat: 2g | Cholesterol: 0mg | Sodium: 33mg | Potassium: 358mg | Fiber: 2g | Sugar: 2g | Vitamin A: 10IU | Vitamin C: 50.7mg | Calcium: 40mg | Iron: 1.1mg

Avocado, Bacon and Balsamic

Perfect for a snack, or even breakfast.

Prep Time: 5 mins

Total Time: 5 mins

Servings: 2 servings

Calories: 254kcal

Ingredients

• 1 avocado

• 2 slices cooked bacon chopped

• 1 teaspoon aged balsamic vinegar to taste

• sea salt to taste

Instructions

1. Halve the avocado and remove pit.

2. Sprinkle with bacon, balsamic vinegar, and sea salt to taste.

3. Serve with a spoon.

Nutrition

Calories: 254kcal | Carbohydrates: 9g | Protein: 4g | Fat: 23g | Saturated Fat: 5g | Cholesterol: 14mg | Sodium: 153mg | Potassium: 530mg | Fiber: 6g | Sugar: 1g | Vitamin A: 145IU | Vitamin C: 10.1mg | Calcium: 12mg | Iron: 0.6mg

Roasted Garlic Baba Ganoush

An easy dip recipe that is gluten-free and paleo-friendly made with the traditional ingredients.

Prep Time: 10 mins

Cook Time: 45 mins

Total Time: 55 mins

Servings: 8 servings

Calories: 88kcal

Ingredients

• 1 head garlic

• 2 medium eggplant

• 3 - 4 tablespoons lemon juice juice of 1-1/2 to 2 lemons

• 2 tablespoons tahini

• 2 tablespoons extra virgin olive oil plus more for drizzling

• ½ teaspoon sea salt

Instructions

1. Preheat oven to 400 degrees.

2. Cut the top off the head of garlic. Place on a sheet of foil and drizzle with olive oil. Wrap tightly in foil and place on a rimmed baking sheet with the eggplants.

3. Roast the vegetables for about 45 minutes, until the eggplants are collapsed and the garlic is completely soft.

4. Cut the eggplants in half lengthwise and place in a colander to cool and drain. Open the garlic packet to cool.

5. Peel the eggplants and squeeze the flesh from the garlic head. Place all ingredients in the food processor and pulse to desired consistency. Taste and adjust seasonings.

Nutrition

Calories: 88kcal | Carbohydrates: 9g | Protein: 2g | Fat: 5g | Saturated Fat: 0g | Cholesterol: 0mg | Sodium: 149mg | Potassium: 300mg | Fiber: 3g |

Sugar: 4g | Vitamin A: 25IU | Vitamin C: 6.3mg | Calcium: 22mg | Iron: 0.5mg

EASY PALEO DINNERS

If you only have a handful of "back pocket" paleo recipes, let them be these ridiculously easy paleo weeknight dinners. These recipes require just a few ingredients, a little hands-on prep time and all can be on the table in 30 minutes or less. Perfect for busy weekday dinners!

Antipasto Salad Recipe

Antipasto salad is an easy no-cook weeknight meal. Gluten-free, grain-free, dairy-free, and paleo - it's perfect when you don't want to turn on the stove.

Prep Time: 10 mins

Total Time: 10 mins

Servings: 3 - 4 servings

Calories: 462kcal

Ingredients

- 1 large head or 2 hearts romaine chopped
- 4 ounces prosciutto cut in strips
- 4 ounces salami or pepperoni cubed
- 1/2 cup artichoke hearts sliced
- 1/2 cup olives mix of black and green

• 1/2 cup hot or sweet peppers pickled or roasted

• Italian dressing to taste

Instructions

1. Combine all ingredients in a large salad bowl. Toss with dressing.

Nutrition

Calories: 462kcal | Carbohydrates: 7g | Protein: 14g | Fat: 41g | Saturated Fat: 11g | Cholesterol: 64mg | Sodium: 1856mg | Potassium: 380mg | Fiber: 3g | Sugar: 2g | Vitamin A: 6000IU | Vitamin C: 20.4mg | Calcium: 57mg | Iron: 1.9mg

Chili Roasted Chicken Thighs

This easy chicken recipe is perfect for quick weeknight dinners.

Prep Time: 5 mins

Cook Time: 15 mins

Total Time: 20 mins

Servings: 8 servings

Calories: 266kcal

Ingredients

• 2 pounds boneless chicken thighs

• 1 tablespoon organic extra virgin olive oil

- 1 tablespoon chili powder

- sea salt to taste

- fresh ground pepper to taste

- fresh cilantro for garnish

- lime wedges for serving

Instructions

1. Preheat oven to 375 degrees.

2. Place chicken on a sheet pan or large baking dish. Drizzle with olive oil and turn to coat. Rub with chili powder, salt, and pepper.

3. Roast the chicken thighs in the oven until cooked through, about 15 minutes.

4. Sprinkle with cilantro and serve with lime wedges.

Nutrition

Calories: 266kcal | Carbohydrates: 0g | Protein: 18g | Fat: 20g | Saturated Fat: 5g | Cholesterol: 111mg | Sodium: 103mg | Potassium: 251mg | Fiber: 0g | Sugar: 0g | Vitamin A: 385IU | Calcium: 12mg | Iron: 0.9mg

Crock Pot Turkey Bolognese Sauce

For an easy weeknight dinner serve this slow cooker turkey Bolognese sauce with zoodles.

Prep Time: 10 mins

Cook Time: 6 hrs

Total Time: 6 hrs 10 mins

Servings: 6 servings

Calories: 231kcal

Ingredients

For sauce

- 1 28- ounce can organic tomato puree
- 1 6- ounce can organic tomato paste
- 1/2 cup chicken stock
- 1 tablespoon olive oil
- 2 teaspoons Italian herb blend
- 1 teaspoon sea salt
- 1/2 teaspoon pepper
- 1/8 teaspoon crushed red pepper flakes
- 3 cloves garlic minced
- 2 small carrots diced
- 1 small onion diced
- 1 pound ground turkey

For zucchini noodles

- 3 - 6 medium zucchini

Instructions

1. Add all sauce ingredients except turkey to slow cooker and stir to combine.

2. Cut ground turkey into cubes, add to slow cooker, and cover with sauce. Do not stir.

3. Cook on low for 6-8 hours.

4. Once the sauce is done, use a potato masher to break up the ground turkey into small chunks.

To make zucchini noodles

1. Spiralize zucchini (1/2 - 1 medium zucchini per serving).

2. Heat one tablespoon olive oil in large frying pan over medium heat. Cook zucchini until warmed through but still firm, about 3 minutes.

Notes

Variations: serve the sauce over roasted spaghetti squash or other spiralized veggie noodles.

Nutrition

Calories: 231kcal | Carbohydrates: 27g | Protein: 24g | Fat: 5g | Cholesterol: 42mg | Sodium: 743mg | Potassium: 1602mg | Fiber: 6g | Sugar: 15g | Vitamin

A: 4840IU | Vitamin C: 49.6mg | Calcium: 84mg | Iron: 4.7mg

Mustard Baked Salmon with Roasted Asparagus

A quick and healthy sheet pan dinner you can have on the table in 15 minutes.

Prep Time: 5 mins

Cook Time: 10 mins

Total Time: 15 mins

Servings: 2 servings

Calories: 336kcal

Ingredients

• 2 salmon fillets (wild caught is best)

• 8 ounces asparagus

• 1 tablespoon garlic infused olive oil

• sea salt to taste

• fresh ground pepper to taste

• 2 tablespoons whole grain mustard to taste

• lemon slices for serving

Instructions

1. Preheat oven to 400 degrees and line a rimmed baking sheet with parchment paper.

2. Put the salmon on one end of the baking sheet and asparagus on the other end. Drizzle asparagus with olive oil and toss to coat. Season with salt and pepper to taste. Spread mustard on top of salmon.

3. Bake until salmon is cooked through and asparagus starts to caramelize but is still crisp, about 10 minutes. Serve with lemon.

Nutrition

Calories: 336kcal | Carbohydrates: 5g | Protein: 36g | Fat: 18g | Saturated Fat: 2g | Cholesterol: 93mg | Sodium: 247mg | Potassium: 1082mg | Fiber: 2g | Sugar: 2g | Vitamin A: 925IU | Vitamin C: 6.4mg | Calcium: 56mg | Iron: 4mg

Garlic Roasted Shrimp with Zucchini Pasta

This easy shrimp with zucchini pasta recipe is a great weeknight dinner — you can have it on the table in 20 minutes.

Prep Time: 10 mins

Cook Time: 10 mins

Total Time: 20 mins

Servings: 2 servings

Calories: 409kcal

Ingredients

• 8 ounces peeled and deveined shrimp thawed if frozen

• 2 tablespoons olive oil

• 2 tablespoons ghee melted (or additional olive oil)

• 2 cloves garlic minced

• 1 lemon zested and juiced

• 1/4 teaspoon salt

• fresh ground pepper to taste

• 2 medium zucchini spiralized or sliced into thin strips for zucchini pasta

Instructions

1. Preheat oven to 400 degrees.

2. Add shrimp, olive oil, ghee, garlic, lemon zest, lemon juice, salt and pepper to the baking dish. Toss to coat shrimp.

3. Bake for 8-10 minutes, turning once. Cook until shrimp are pink and just cooked through, or until heated through if using pre-cooked shrimp.

4. Add the zucchini pasta, toss and serve.

Nutrition

Calories: 409kcal | Carbohydrates: 8g | Protein: 25g | Fat: 31g | Saturated Fat: 11g | Cholesterol: 324mg |

Sodium: 1188mg | Potassium: 602mg | Fiber: 1g | Sugar: 5g | Vitamin A: 390IU | Vitamin C: 46.4mg | Calcium: 201mg | Iron: 3.1mg

Easy Paleo Smoothie Recipes

These quick and easy paleo smoothie recipes are all dairy-free and deliciously simple. Try a smoothie for breakfast—they make your mornings so much easier when you're on-the-go!

Paleo Strawberry Coconut Smoothie

This paleo strawberry coconut smoothie is sweet and creamy with no added sugar or dairy.

Prep Time: 5 mins

Total Time: 5 mins

Servings: 2 servings

Calories: 346kcal

Ingredients

- 1 cup coconut milk

- 1 frozen banana sliced

- 2 cups frozen strawberries

- 1 teaspoon vanilla extract

- 1 scoop collagen protein powder optional

Instructions

1. Add all ingredients to high-speed blender and blend until smooth.

Calories: 346kcal | Carbohydrates: 27g | Protein: 8g | Fat: 24g | Saturated Fat: 21g | Sodium: 40mg | Potassium: 680mg | Fiber: 4g | Sugar: 14g | Vitamin A: 40IU | Vitamin C: 90.9mg | Calcium: 43mg | Iron: 4.5mg

3-Ingredient Green Smoothie Recipe

Just 3 Ingredientsand this spinach green smoothie tastes like a pina colada!

Prep Time: 5 mins

Total Time: 5 mins

Servings: 2 serving

Calories: 211kcal

Ingredients

- 1 cup fresh baby spinach
- 3/4 cup coconut milk
- 1 cup frozen pineapple

Instructions

1. Add coconut milk and spinach to blender. Blend on high speed until completely smooth.

2. Add frozen pineapple and blend again, until smooth.

Calories: 211kcal | Carbohydrates: 13g | Protein: 2g | Fat: 18g | Saturated Fat: 16g | Cholesterol: 0mg | Sodium: 23mg | Potassium: 360mg | Fiber: 1g | Sugar: 8g | Vitamin A: 1455IU | Vitamin C: 44.5mg| Calcium: 41mg | Iron: 3.4mg

Peach Coconut Milk Smoothie

A delicious dairy-free peaches and cream smoothie with just 4 ingredients.

Prep Time: 10 mins

Total Time: 10 mins

Servings: 3 servings

Calories: 187kcal

Ingredients

• 1 cup coconut milk chilled

• 1 cup ice

• 2 fresh peaches peeled and cut into chunks

• lemon zest to taste

Instructions

1. Add coconut milk, ice and peaches to Vitamix or blender. Using a microplane, add a few gratings of fresh lemon zest, to taste.

2. Blend on high speed until smooth.

Nutrition

Calories: 187kcal | Carbohydrates: 12g | Protein: 2g | Fat: 16g | Saturated Fat: 14g | Sodium: 10mg | Potassium: 356mg | Fiber: 2g | Sugar: 8g | Vitamin A: 325IU | Vitamin C: 7.3mg | Calcium: 20mg | Iron: 2.7mg

Paleo Key Lime Pie Smoothie

An easy paleo key lime smoothie recipe with avocado and coconut milk.

Prep Time: 5 mins

Total Time: 5 mins

Servings: 3 servings

Calories: 242kcal

Ingredients

- 1 cup coconut milk

- 1 cup ice

- 1/2 avocado

- zest and juice of 2 limes

- stevia, local raw honey, maple syrup or sweetener of choice, to taste

Instructions

1. Add coconut milk, ice, avocado, lime zest, lime juice, and honey to Vitamix or blender. Blend until smooth.

Nutrition

Calories: 242kcal | Carbohydrates: 8g | Protein: 2g | Fat: 23g | Saturated Fat: 17g | Cholesterol: 0mg | Sodium: 14mg | Potassium: 396mg | Fiber: 4g | Sugar: 3g | Vitamin A: 50IU | Vitamin C: 11.6mg | Calcium: 17mg | Iron: 1.5mg

Pumpkin Coconut Smoothie Recipe

A smoothie version of pumpkin pie that's paleo, vegan, and dairy-free!

Prep Time: 5 mins

Total Time: 5 mins

Servings: 2 servings

Calories: 292kcal

Ingredients

• 1 cup coconut milk

• 1/4 cup organic pumpkin puree

• 2 teaspoons pumpkin pie spice (can substitute cinnamon and ginger)

- 1 frozen banana sliced (omit for keto version)
- 1 cup ice

Instructions

1. Add coconut milk, pumpkin, pumpkin pie spice, banana, and ice to Blendtec or Vitamix.

2. Blend on smoothie cycle or high speed until smooth.

Nutrition

Calories: 292kcal | Carbohydrates: 20g | Protein: 3g | Fat: 24g | Saturated Fat: 21g | Sodium: 18mg | Potassium: 522mg | Fiber: 2g | Sugar: 8g | Vitamin A: 4805IU | Vitamin C: 8mg | Calcium: 42mg | Iron: 4.7mg

Healthy Shamrock Shake Recipe

Made with coconut milk, avocado, and fresh mint, this healthy shamrock shake recipe lets you indulge without all the scary ingredients.

Prep Time: 5 mins

Total Time: 5 mins

Servings: 2 servings

Calories: 308kcal

Ingredients

• 1 cup coconut milk

• 1 cup ice

• 1/2 avocado

• 1 teaspoon organic vanilla extract

• 1 large handful fresh mint leaves to taste

• stevia, local raw honey, or maple syrup to taste

Instructions

1. Add all ingredients to the blender and blend until smooth.

Nutrition

Calories: 308kcal | Carbohydrates: 7g | Protein: 3g | Fat: 31g | Saturated Fat: 22g | Sodium: 18mg | Potassium: 492mg | Fiber: 3g | Vitamin A: 75IU | Vitamin C: 6.2mg | Calcium: 26mg | Iron: 4mg

Espresso Protein Shake

This espresso protein shake is creamy and thick like a frozen coffee shop drink.

Prep Time: 5 mins

Total Time: 5 mins

Servings: 1 serving

Ingredients

- 1/2 cup cashew milk
- 1/2 banana frozen
- 2/3 cup ice cubes
- 1/2 teaspoon vanilla extract
- dash of cinnamon
- 1/4 cup unflavored egg white protein powder
- 2 ounces espresso or strong coffee
- honey or sweetener of choice optional

Instructions

1. Add all Ingredientsto Vitamix and blend on high until smooth. Pour into a tall glass and serve.

Paleo Chocolate Coconut Smoothie

A rich and creamy, chocolate smoothie with no dairy or added sugar.

Prep Time: 5 mins

Total Time: 5 mins

Servings: 2 servings

Calories: 160kcal

Ingredients

- 1 cup coconut milk
- 1 frozen banana sliced

- 1 cup ice
- 1/4 cup raw cacao powder
- 1 scoop collagen protein powder

Instructions

1. Add all Ingredientsto Vitamix or high power blender and blend until smooth.

Nutrition

Calories: 160kcal | Carbohydrates: 23g | Protein: 2g | Fat: 8g | Saturated Fat: 7g | Cholesterol: 0mg | Sodium: 86mg | Potassium: 375mg | Fiber: 5g | Sugar: 7g | Vitamin A: 40IU | Vitamin C: 5.1mg | Calcium: 14mg | Iron: 1.6mg

Paleo Banana Bread Smoothie

A simple smoothie that tastes like banana bread!

Prep Time: 5 mins

Total Time: 5 mins

Servings: 2 servings

Calories: 237kcal

Ingredients

- 1 cup cashew milk
- 2 frozen bananas sliced
- 2 tablespoons almond butter

• fresh ground nutmeg to taste

• collagen protein powder (optional)

Instructions

1. Combine all Ingredientsin high-speed blender and blend until sooth.

2. Garnish with fresh nutmeg.

Notes

For vegan or vegetarian: omit collagen powder or substitute vegan protein powder.

Nutrition

Calories: 237kcal | Carbohydrates: 30g | Protein: 10g | Fat: 10g | Saturated Fat: 1g | Sodium: 100mg | Potassium: 542mg | Fiber: 5g | Sugar: 15g | Vitamin A: 76IU | Vitamin C: 10mg | Calcium: 61mg | Iron: 1mg

Paleo Pina Colada Smoothie

This paleo pina colada smoothie is pure tropical simplicity.

Prep Time: 5 mins

Total Time: 5 mins

Servings: 1 serving

Ingredients

• 3/4 cup coconut milk

• 3/4 cup frozen pineapple

Instructions

1. Add all ingredients to Vitamix in order listed and blend on high until smooth. Pour into a tall glass and serve.

CONCLUSION

Thank you so much for choosing to pick up this book on the Paleo Diet. We hope that you enjoyed the information and that it benefitted you in more ways than one. We know that weight loss and being fit can be a troubling time, this is exactly why we wanted to inform you on every aspect of this diet to equip you with the proper tools. You are now ready to go take the world on produce the results to create those brighter days!